# STOP DREAMING

## Accept Yourself As You Are

Dr. ANDREA SCARSI

# DESCRIPTION

Stop Dreaming and Accept Yourself as You Are.

Do you ever feel like you need to be better? Do you need to live up to your potential? If so, you're not alone. Many people struggle with feelings of inadequacy and self-doubt. But what if I told you you don't have to be perfect? What if I told you that you can be happy and prosperous like you are?

In this book, I will show you how to stop dreaming and start living in the present moment. I will guide you on accepting yourself for who you are and your flaws. And I will show you how to live a life full of joy and fulfillment.

If you're ready to stop dreaming and accept yourself as you are, this book is for you.

We'll explore The Problem with Dreaming.

We all dream. We dream about the future, about what we want to be and what we want to achieve. But sometimes, our dreams get in the way of our happiness.

We're not living in the present moment when we constantly dream about the future. We're not enjoying the here and now. We're always looking ahead to the next thing: goal and achievement.

This leads to more stress and anxiety. We're never satisfied with what we have. We're always striving for more. And this takes a toll on our mental and emotional health.

So, what to do about it? How do we stop dreaming and start accepting ourselves?

The first step is to become aware of your dreams. What are you dreaming about? What are you hoping to achieve? Once you're aware of your dreams, you challenge them.

**Ask yourself**: Are these dreams really what I want? Or are they what I should want?

Are these dreams realistic? Or are they pipe dreams?

Are these dreams making me happy? Or are they making me stressed and anxious?

Once you've challenged your dreams, you start to let them go. You begin to focus on the present moment and enjoy what you have.

We'll explore Accepting Yourself.

One of the biggest obstacles to happiness is not accepting yourself for who you are. We all have flaws and imperfections. But we must learn to accept these flaws and imperfections as part of our identity.

When we don't accept ourselves, we constantly try to change ourselves. We're trying to be someone we're not. And this leads to much unhappiness.

So, how do we learn to accept ourselves?

The first step is to be kind to yourself. Forgive yourself for your mistakes. Accept your flaws and imperfections.

The second step is to focus on your strengths. What are you good at? What do you like about yourself?

The third step is to surround yourself with positive people. People who love and accept you for who you are.

When you learn to accept yourself, you'll be free to live a happy and fulfilling life.

We'll explore Living in the Present Moment.

The key to happiness is living in the present moment. We're not enjoying the here and now when constantly worrying about the future or regretting the past.

So, how do we learn to live in the present moment?

The first step is to be mindful. Pay attention to your thoughts and feelings. Notice when you're getting caught up in the past or the future.

The second step is to focus on your breath. When you focus on your breath, you return to the present moment.

The third step is to practice gratitude. When you focus on the things you're grateful for, you're more likely to appreciate the present moment.

When you learn to live in the present moment, you'll be free to experience life's joy and happiness.

In conclusion, before moving to the book, stop dreaming and accept yourself for who you are. And start living in the present moment. When you do these things, you'll be free to experience life's joy and happiness.

DEDICATED

To Those Wanting To Feel Good About Themselves

# TABLE OF CONTENTS

# ACKNOWLEDGMENTS

I thank all those who constantly remind me that
I'm okay as I am.

# NOTE OF THE AUTHOR

The Author strived to be accurate and complete when creating this book. Nevertheless, he affirms that the contents expressed in it are solely the result of his knowledge, experience, and competence in the considered discipline and does not guarantee and declare at any time that these are absolute and unequivocal.

While he made all attempts to verify the information in this publication, he assumes no responsibility for errors, omissions, different interpretations, or experimentations of the subject matter herein.

Any perceived slights of specific persons, peoples, companies, or organizations are unintentional.

There are no guarantees of performed results or income made in self-help books and manuals, as one expects. Readers must rely on their judgment about any single circumstance and act accordingly.

This book does not pretend to be an official medical, dietetic, psychological, religious, legal, commercial, accounting, or financial professional source. The Readers must seek the services of competent professionals in all the abovementioned fields.

Enjoy.

ANDREA SCARSI

# THE POWER OF AWARENESS

Understanding Your True Self.

Understanding Your True Self is a crucial step in the journey of self-awareness. It involves looking deep within yourself to discover yourself beyond the masks and facades you have adopted over the years. Many of us go through life not truly knowing ourselves, constantly seeking validation and approval from others. However, true fulfillment and happiness only come from accepting and embracing our true selves.

For those on a path of self-discovery, it is essential to take the time to reflect on your values, beliefs, passions, and desires. What makes you unique? What brings you joy and fulfillment? Understanding your true self aligns your actions and goals with your authentic self, leading to a more purposeful and fulfilling life.

Dreamers often have a deep connection to their inner selves. Still, even they benefit from further exploration and understanding. Through meditation and dream analysis, you uncover hidden aspects of your true self and gain insights into your subconscious mind.

Network marketers, who often focus on building connections with others, also benefit from understanding their true selves. Being authentic and genuine to yourself attracts like-minded individuals and builds more genuine and meaningful relationships.

It is easy to lose sight of who we are in a world that constantly bombards us with images of perfection and success. However, by taking the time to understand and accept yourself as you are, you unlock your true potential and live a more fulfilling and authentic life. Embrace your true self, stop dreaming, and start living your truth.

Embracing Your Flaws and Imperfections.

In the journey of self-awareness, one of the most critical steps is learning to embrace your flaws and imperfections. It is essential to understand that no one is perfect, and we all have unique strengths and weaknesses. By accepting and embracing our flaws, we cultivate a more profound sense of self-compassion and self-love.

For many people, the idea of embracing their flaws is challenging. Society often pressures us to be perfect, leading to feelings of inadequacy and low self-esteem. However, accurate self-awareness comes from accepting ourselves as we are, flaws and all. By acknowledging and embracing our imperfections, we relinquish the need for external validation and find true happiness within ourselves.

Dreamers often struggle with self-acceptance, as they may have high expectations for themselves and their spiritual growth. However, true enlightenment comes from accepting ourselves completely, flaws and all. By embracing our imperfections, we let go of self-judgment and cultivate a more profound inner peace.

For network marketers, embracing flaws and

imperfections is a powerful and compassionate tool for building authentic connections with others. We create genuine relationships based on trust and mutual understanding by showing vulnerability and humility. People are drawn to authenticity; we inspire others to do the same by embracing our flaws.

In conclusion, embracing your flaws and imperfections is essential to self-awareness. By accepting yourself as you are, you cultivate a more profound sense of self-compassion, self-love, and authenticity. Remember, you are perfectly imperfect, which makes you truly unique. Stop dreaming of perfection and start living your most authentic life.

Letting Go of Self-Doubt.

Letting go of self-doubt is a crucial step on the journey to self-awareness. To start living and embrace who you are, you must release the negative beliefs and limitations that hold you back. Self-doubt is a toxic force that prevents you from reaching your full potential and living your desired life.

For those on a path of self-discovery and seeking truth, letting go of self-doubt is necessary. Through meditation and introspection, you identify the root causes of your self-doubt and work towards overcoming them. By acknowledging and accepting yourself as you are, you build a foundation of self-love and confidence to navigate life's challenges with grace and resilience.

For the dreamers and network marketers, letting go of self-doubt is essential for achieving success and reaching your goals. Believing in yourself and your abilities is the first step towards manifesting your dreams and creating your desired life. By letting go of self-doubt, you open yourself to endless possibilities and great opportunities for growth and transformation.

In the journey to self-awareness, it is essential to remember that self-doubt is a natural part of the human experience. However, it is also overcome with dedication, perseverance, and a determined willingness to confront your fears and insecurities head-on. By letting go of self-doubt and embracing who you are with love and acceptance, you genuinely stop dreaming and start living the life you were meant to live.

# BREAKING FREE FROM LIMITING BELIEFS

Identifying Your Limiting Beliefs.

To truly begin the journey to self-awareness and start living the life of your dreams, it is essential to first identify and address your limiting beliefs. These negative thought patterns and beliefs keep you from reaching your full potential and living your desired life.

For many of us, these limiting beliefs are deeply ingrained in our subconscious minds, making them difficult to recognize and overcome. However, by exploring and identifying these beliefs, you break free from their hold and create a new, empowering mindset.

One way to identify your limiting beliefs is to pay attention to the negative self-talk in your mind. Notice when you doubt, criticize, or tell yourself you are not good enough. These are all indications of underlying limiting beliefs that are holding you back.

Another helpful exercise is to think about the areas where you feel stuck or unable to progress. This could be in your career, relationships, health, or any other aspect of your life. Examining these areas uncovers the limiting beliefs keeping you from moving forward.

As you identify your limiting beliefs, it is essential to remember that you are not defined by them. They are thoughts and beliefs you change and replace with more positive and empowering ones. You begin to reprogram your mind and let go of these limiting beliefs through meditation, self-reflection, and affirmations.

By taking the time to identify and address your limiting beliefs, you clear the path to self-awareness and start living the life you truly desire. Remember, you change your thoughts and beliefs, creating a life filled with joy, purpose, empathy, and fulfillment.

Challenging Negative Thought Patterns.

One of the biggest obstacles we face in the quest for self-awareness is challenging negative thought patterns. These destructive patterns keep us from reaching our full potential and living fulfilling lives. Let's explore strategies to identify and overcome these negative thoughts to stop dreaming and start living.

Negative thought patterns manifest in various ways, such as self-doubt, fear of failure, or limiting beliefs about ourselves. These thoughts create a cycle of negativity that keeps us stuck in a state of inaction and prevents us from taking steps toward our goals. By becoming aware of these patterns, we challenge and change them.

One effective strategy for challenging negative thought patterns is mindfulness and meditation. Practicing mindfulness, we observe our thoughts without judgment and recognize when negative patterns arise. Through meditation, we cultivate a sense of inner peace and clarity that lets us let go of these destructive thoughts.

Another powerful tool for challenging negative thought

patterns is positive affirmations. By replacing negative self-talk with positive affirmations, we rewire our brains to focus on the good rather than the bad. Affirmations help us build self-confidence, overcome limiting beliefs, and shift our mindset towards a more joyful and positive outlook.

Addressing and challenging negative thought patterns is essential for those searching for truth and seeking to stop dreaming and start living. By practicing mindfulness, meditation, and positive affirmations, we take control of our thoughts and emotions and create a present life filled with purpose, fulfillment, and delight. Remember, you have the power to change your thoughts and change your life. Embrace self-acceptance and believe in yourself as you are.

Cultivating a Growth Mindset.

Cultivating a Growth Mindset is essential for anyone on the path to self-awareness and personal growth. Let's explore the power of adopting a growth mindset and how it positively impacts all areas of your life.

A growth mindset is the certainty that one's abilities and intelligence develop through hard work, dedication, and perseverance. This mindset starkly contrasts with a fixed mindset, which believes that abilities are predetermined and unchangeable.

For those on a journey of self-awareness, cultivating a growth mindset is crucial. It allows us to embrace and learn from challenges and failures and see setbacks as the best opportunities for growth. By adopting a growth mindset, you overcome limiting beliefs and self-doubt and begin to unleash your full potential.

Dreamers, network marketers, and anyone searching for truth benefit significantly from developing a growth mindset. You create your desired life by shifting your perspective from limitations to possibilities.

Let's now explore practical strategies for cultivating a growth mindset, including:

1. Embracing challenges and viewing them as opportunities for growth.

2. Learning from failures and setbacks rather than allowing them to define you.

3. Seeking out feedback to improve and grow.

4. Cultivating a sense of curiosity and a willingness to learn new things.

By adopting a growth mindset, you stop dreaming and start living the life you were meant to live. Accept yourself as you are while believing in your ability to grow and evolve into the best version of yourself. All this empowers you to take control of your life now and create your desired future.

# THE ART OF MINDFULNESS

Practicing Mindful Awareness.

Practicing mindful awareness is a powerful tool for those seeking to deepen their understanding of themselves and their world. By bringing conscious attention to our thoughts, emotions, sensations, and sentiments in the present moment, we cultivate a sense of clarity, peace, and connection to our inner selves.

Mindful awareness offers a pathway to self-discovery and personal growth for general individuals or people searching for truth. By becoming more attuned to our thoughts, presumptions, and feelings without judgment, we unravel the layers of conditioning and limiting beliefs that hold us back from living authentically. Through mindfulness meditation, breathwork, and body scanning, we learn to observe our inner world with curiosity and compassion, gaining valuable insights into our true nature and desires.

For dreamers, mindful awareness enhances the depth and quality of their practice. They access deeper states of consciousness and insight by bringing a sense of focused attention and presence to their meditations or dream explorations. Mindful awareness also helps dreamers become more lucid, allowing them to consciously navigate and interact with the dream environment.

For network marketers or those in the self-help niche, practicing mindful awareness improves their ability to connect with others authentically and cultivate meaningful relationships. They build trust, rapport, and empathy with their clients and colleagues by approaching their interactions with presence, compassion, and active listening. Mindful awareness also helps them stay grounded and focused amidst the distractions and pressures of their work, allowing them to make more informed decisions and take purposeful action toward their goals.

In conclusion, practicing mindful awareness is a transformative practice that benefits individuals from all walks of life. By incorporating it into our daily routines and interactions, we cultivate greater self-awareness, acceptance, and connection to the world around us. Stop dreaming and start living by embracing the power of mindful awareness today.

Living in the Present Moment.
Living in the present moment is often discussed in self-help books, meditation practices, and spiritual teachings. But what does it indeed mean to live in the present moment? And why is it so crucial for our overall well-being and personal growth?

Living in the present moment means being fully aware and engaged in what is happening without dwelling on the past or worrying about the future. It means accepting and embracing the reality of the present moment, no matter how challenging or uncomfortable it may be. By living in the present moment, we let go of regrets, fears, and anxieties that hold us back from living our lives to the fullest.

Living in the present moment is a powerful practice for those constantly dreaming and planning for the future. It allows us to appreciate the beauty and wonder of life happening right now instead of continually chasing after a future that may never come to fruition. By living in the present moment, we fully experience the joy, peace, and contentment available to us in each moment.

For network marketers, living in the present moment is particularly beneficial. By focusing on the present moment, we are more attentive and responsive to the needs of our clients and customers. We are also more present and engaged in our interactions, building more powerful and authentic relationships.

In conclusion, living in the present moment is a powerful practice that brings us greater peace, happiness, and fulfillment. By letting go of the past and future and embracing the present moment's reality, we live our lives to the fullest. So let go of your dreams and fears and start living in the present moment today.

Finding Peace Through Meditation.
In the chaotic and fast-paced world we live in, finding inner peace seems like an impossible task. However, meditation teaches us to quiet our minds, connect with our inner selves, and find the peace we desperately seek. Let's then explore the power of this ancient practice and how it transforms our lives.

Meditation is not just about sitting silently for a few minutes each day. It is a powerful tool that helps us to calm our minds, reduce stress, and increase our self-awareness. Meditating teaches us to let go of negative thoughts and emotions while cultivating inner peace that will stay with us throughout the day.

Meditation is a game-changer for those constantly chasing their dreams and never pausing and reflecting. Incorporating this practice into your everyday routine teaches you to quiet the outside world's noise and connect with your true self. This leads to greater clarity, purpose, and fulfillment.

Whether you are a seasoned meditator or someone just beginning to explore this practice, finding peace through meditation is possible for everyone. By dedicating just a few minutes each day, up to one hour, to quieting your mind and emotions and connecting with your inner self, you experience profound changes in your life. So, stop dreaming and start living by embracing the power of meditation to find the peace and contentment you have been searching for.

# SETTING GOALS AND TAKING ACTIONS

Defining Your Life Purpose.

To indeed start living a fulfilling life, it is crucial to first define your life purpose. This drives your actions and decisions, guiding you towards a life of meaning and fulfillment. With a clear understanding of your purpose, you may feel safe and fulfilled, constantly searching for something more.

To define your life purpose, reflect on what truly matters to you. What brings you joy and fulfillment? What are your values and beliefs? What are you passionate about? These are all critical questions to consider when trying to determine your purpose.

Meditation is a powerful tool for those searching for truth and uncovering your true purpose. By quieting your mind and tuning into your inner self, you gain clarity and insight into what you are meant to do in this world. Meditation helps you connect directly with your higher self and tap into the wisdom within you.

For dreamers and network marketers, defining your life purpose helps you stay focused and motivated as you work towards your goals. Knowing your purpose gives you a sense of direction and drive, allowing you to overcome obstacles and remain committed to your vision.

In the journey to self-awareness, defining your life purpose is crucial to living a fulfilling and meaningful life. Take the time to reflect on what truly matters to you, and let that guide you towards a life of purpose and passion. Stop dreaming and start living the life you were meant to live.

Creating a Vision Board.

Creating a vision board is a powerful yet simple tool that helps you manifest your dreams and goals into reality. Whether you want to improve relationships, advance your career, or enhance your well-being, a vision board visually represents your aspirations and desires.

To create a vision board, gather materials from magazines, newspapers, photographs, quotes, and images that resonate with your goals and aspirations. You also incorporate personal items such as drawings, affirmations, and mementos that hold special meaning to you.

Once you have collected your materials, find a quiet and peaceful space to focus on your intentions. Take a few moments to center yourself through meditation, breathing exercises, or chanting to clear your mind and set a positive tone for the creative process.

Begin by organizing your materials and selecting images and words that reflect your deepest desires and aspirations. Arrange them on a board in a way that feels visually appealing and inspiring to you. To create a more structured vision board, you also categorize your goals into different sections: career, relationships, health, and personal growth.

As you continue to build your vision board, allow yourself to dream big and envision the life you truly desire. Visualize yourself already living the life of your dreams and feel joy, gratitude, and fulfillment as if your goals have already been achieved.

By creating a vision board, you set clear intentions for your future and activate the power of attraction to bring your desires into your reality. Keep your vision board where you see it daily to stay motivated and inspired on your journey toward self-awareness and personal growth. Remember, the power lies within you to stop dreaming and start living the life you truly deserve.

Developing an Action Plan.

Developing an action plan is crucial for self-awareness and personal growth. Creating a roadmap towards your goals and aspirations is essential to stop dreaming and start living. Let's then provide practical tips on developing an action plan tailored to your unique needs and circumstances.

First and foremost, setting clear, specific, and big goals for yourself is essential. Take the time to reflect on what you truly want to achieve in life and write down your objectives in a journal or diary. Whether you aspire to improve your relationships, advance your career, or enhance your overall well-being, having a clear vision of your goals will help you stay focused and motivated.

Next, break down your goals into smaller and manageable tasks that you tackle one step at a time, each within a specific time. Consider creating a timeline or schedule to keep track of your progress and hold yourself accountable. Remember to celebrate your achievements, no matter how small they seem.

Additionally, identify potential obstacles or challenges as you work towards your goals. Develop strategies for overcoming these hurdles, and be prepared to adjust your action plan as needed. Stay open-minded, flexible, and willing to seek support from others when necessary.

In conclusion, developing an action plan is critical to self-awareness and personal growth. Setting clear goals to complete within a specific time, breaking them down into manageable tasks, and anticipating obstacles create a roadmap to help you turn your dreams into reality. Remember, the journey towards self-acceptance and fulfillment starts with taking the first step.

# BUILDING RESILIENCE AND OVERCOMING OBSTACLES

Embracing Failure as a Learning Opportunity

In our journey to self-awareness, we must learn to embrace failure and criticism as valuable learning opportunities. Failure is not something to be feared or avoided; it is a necessary step toward growth and success. When we allow ourselves to make mistakes and learn from them, we open ourselves up to new possibilities and a deeper understanding of ourselves.

For many of us, failure is a source of shame and embarrassment. We may have let ourselves down or need to fulfill our full potential. However, it is crucial to remember that failure is a natural part of life and a valuable teacher. Failure is necessary for us to learn and grow. We would never discover our strengths and weaknesses or uncover our true potential.

Dreamers and network marketers must learn to see and accept failure as a stepping stone to success. Each failure is an opportunity to learn more about ourselves and our goals. It is a chance to reassess our strategies, set new intentions, and move forward with renewed determination.

By embracing failure as a joyful learning opportunity, we cultivate a growth mindset and develop the resilience needed to quickly overcome any obstacles that come our way. We learn to accept ourselves as we are, imperfections and all, and move forward with confidence and self-assurance.

So, let us stop dreaming and start living by embracing failure as a valuable teacher on our journey to self-awareness. Let us learn from our mistakes, grow from our setbacks, and ultimately, become the best versions of ourselves.

Cultivating Self-Compassion.

Cultivating self-compassion is a crucial step to self-awareness and personal growth. Practicing self-compassion in a world that often emphasizes self-criticism and perfectionism is challenging. However, it is essential for our mental well-being and overall happiness.

Self-compassion means treating ourselves with the same kindness, respect, and understanding we would offer a lover or a close friend. It means acknowledging our flaws and imperfections without judgment and accepting ourselves as we are now. By cultivating self-compassion, we learn to be more forgiving, leading to greater self-acceptance and a more positive self-image.

One way to cultivate self-compassion is through mindfulness and meditation. By practicing mindfulness, we become aware of our train of thoughts and deep feelings and learn to observe them without attaching judgment. This helps us to develop a more compassionate attitude towards ourselves as we learn to accept our thoughts and emotions without criticism.

Another way to cultivate self-compassion is to practice self-care and self-love. This involves taking time for yourself, engaging in activities that bring you joy, and treating yourself with kindness and respect. By prioritizing self-care, you nurture a sense of compassion toward yourself, positively impacting your overall well-being.

In conclusion, cultivating self-compassion is a mighty personal growth and self-awareness tool. We develop a more positive relationship with ourselves and others by learning to treat ourselves with kindness, respect, and understanding. So, stop dreaming and start living by embracing self-compassion and accepting yourself as you are.


Finding Strength in Adversity.

Life consists of challenges and obstacles that sometimes make us feel defeated or hopeless. However, we experiment with our inner strength and resilience during these difficult times. Let's explore how adversity catalyzes personal growth and self-awareness.

For those constantly dreaming and seeking fulfillment, facing adversity feels like a setback or a roadblock. But what if we reframed our perspective and saw adversity as an opportunity for growth and transformation? We discover our true strength and potential by embracing challenges and obstacles.

Dreamers understand the power of the mind and the importance of staying present in the moment. When faced with adversity, it is crucial to stay grounded and centered, using mindfulness and meditation practices to navigate complex emotions and situations. By staying connected to our inner selves, we find the positive strength to overcome any adversity that comes our way.

Network marketers are no strangers to rejection and setbacks. In fact, they understand that failure is simply a part of the journey to success. By embracing adversity and learning from our mistakes, we become more resilient and adaptable when facing challenges.

Ultimately, finding strength in adversity requires us to accept ourselves as we are, flaws and all. By acknowledging our weaknesses and vulnerabilities, we tap into the most bottomless well of inner strength and courage. All this guides you on a journey of self-discovery and empowerment, helping you to stop dreaming and start living a life of purpose and fulfillment.

# CULTIVATING POSITIVE RELATIONSHIPS

Surrounding Yourself with Supportive People.

In our journey to self-awareness, one of the most critical factors that significantly impact our growth is the people we surround ourselves with. It is crucial to be mindful of the energy and influence that others bring into our lives, as they either uplift us or hold us back from reaching our full potential.

A solid support system is essential for those of us on a path of self-discovery and personal development. Surrounding yourself with supportive people who believe in your dreams and encourage you to be your best version makes all the difference in your journey.

Dreamers understand the power of positive energy and the importance of cultivating a peaceful and harmonious environment. By surrounding yourself with like-minded people who share your values and beliefs, you create a space that nurtures your spiritual growth and helps you stay aligned with your true purpose.

Dreamers often face skepticism and doubt from others who may not understand their vision or passions. By surrounding yourself with supportive people who share your enthusiasm for dreaming big and taking risks, you find the courage and motivation to pursue your goals confidently.

Network marketers know the value of building solid relationships and connections with others. By surrounding yourself with supportive mentors, colleagues, and friends who believe in your potential and are willing to help you succeed, you expand your reach and achieve tremendous success in your business endeavors.

In self-help and personal growth, accepting yourself as you are is critical to finding inner peace and fulfillment. Surrounding yourself with supportive people who accept you unconditionally and empower you to embrace your true self helps you build confidence and self-love.

Remember, the people you surround yourself with either lift or bring you down. Choose wisely and surround yourself with those who support your journey to self-awareness and help you become the best version of yourself.

Setting Boundaries with Toxic Individuals.

In our journey to self-awareness, we must recognize and address toxic individuals. These people drain our energy, manipulate us, and bring negativity into our world. Setting boundaries with poisonous individuals is crucial for our mental and emotional well-being.

Toxic individuals come in many forms - from friends and family members to colleagues and acquaintances. They exhibit behaviors such as constant criticism, gaslighting, or passive-aggressiveness. Identifying these individuals and protecting ourselves from their harmful influence is essential.

One way to set boundaries with toxic individuals is to limit our interactions. It means avoiding specific social gatherings or limiting communication to essential matters only. It is also important to communicate clearly and assertively about what behaviors are unacceptable to us.

Another important aspect of setting boundaries with toxic individuals is to prioritize self-care. It involves practicing mindfulness and self-love, engaging in joyous activities, and surrounding ourselves with positive and supportive people. By taking care of ourselves, we are better equipped to deal with toxic individuals and their negative impact on our lives.

As we continue our journey to self-awareness, it is essential to remember that we choose who we allow into our lives. By setting boundaries with toxic individuals, we take a proactive step and start creating a healthy and positive environment for ourselves. Remember, putting yourself first and prioritizing your well-being above all else is okay.

Practicing Empathy and Compassion.

Practicing empathy and compassion is a crucial step on the journey to self-awareness. Cultivating these qualities in our daily lives is more important than ever in a world that often feels divided and disconnected. By understanding and sharing the feelings of others, we build deeper connections and foster a sense of unity within ourselves and our communities.

Empathy is the mastery of genuinely putting oneself in someone else's shoes to experience their perspective. It requires active listening, without judgment, and responding with kindness and understanding. Conversely, compassion is the desire to alleviate other's suffering and to show care and concern for their well-being. Empathy and compassion form the foundation of a more compassionate and understanding world.

For those on a journey of self-discovery and personal growth, practicing empathy and compassion is a powerful tool for transformation. By opening our hearts to the experiences of others, we learn more about ourselves and our own emotions. This increased awareness helps us to navigate our struggles and challenges with greater ease and understanding.

For dreamers and network marketers, cultivating empathy and compassion also has tangible benefits. By developing a deeper comprehension of the needs and desires of others, we build stronger relationships and create more meaningful connections. It leads to increased success in our personal and professional lives and a greater sense of fulfillment and purpose.

Empathy and compassion stand in meditation as essential qualities to cultivate. By quieting the mind and turning our attention inward, we develop greater empathy for ourselves and others, which leads to a more peaceful and harmonious existence, both internally and externally.

In conclusion, practicing empathy and compassion is beneficial for our relationships and personal growth and essential for creating a more compassionate and understanding world. By embracing these qualities daily, we move closer to our true selves and create a more harmonious and fulfilling existence.

# LIVING AUTHENTICALLY
# AND FULFILLING YOUR POTENTIAL

Honoring Your Values and Beliefs.

Let's explore the importance of honoring your values and beliefs to live a fulfilling and authentic life. As individuals on a journey to self-awareness, it is crucial to understand what truly matters to us and to stay true to ourselves despite external pressures and expectations.

Our values and beliefs shape our identity and guide our decisions and actions. They are the foundation of who we are and what we stand for. When we align our thoughts, words, and deeds with our core values, we experience a sense of inner peace and fulfillment. On the other hand, when we compromise our values for the sake of others or societal norms, we feel disconnected from ourselves and experience inner turmoil.

As dreamers and seekers of truth, we must regularly reflect on our values and beliefs. Take the time to identify what is truly important to you and what you hold dear. We do it through introspection, meditation, or journaling. By getting in touch with your innermost desires and convictions, you gain clarity on what you want out of life and how you want to show up in the world.

For network marketers, honoring your values and beliefs is also a powerful tool for building authentic connections. People are more likely to trust and resonate with you when you are true to yourself and your values, which leads to deeper and more meaningful personal and professional relationships.

In conclusion, honoring your values and beliefs is critical to self-awareness and personal growth. You live a more purposeful and fulfilling life by staying true to yourself and your beliefs. Embrace who you are, accept yourself as you are, and let your values guide your journey to stop dreaming and start living.

Expressing Your True Self.

In a world filled with expectations and societal pressures, losing sight of who we are is effortless. We often find ourselves conforming to the norms and standards others set instead of embracing our authentic selves. However, expressing your true self is the key to living a fulfilling and meaningful life.

Expressing our true selves taps into our innermost desires, passions, and values and allows us to live authentically and in alignment with our true purpose. By embracing who we are and expressing ourselves genuinely, we open ourselves to endless possibilities and opportunities.

Expressing your true self is essential for those on a journey of self-awareness. It is about accepting yourself as you are, flaws and all, and allowing yourself to shine uniquely. This process is liberating and empowering, as it enables you to break free from the constraints of societal expectations and embrace your individuality.

Dreamers often understand the importance of expressing their true selves. Through meditation and visualization, they connect with their innermost selves and uncover their deepest desires and aspirations. By expressing their true selves, they manifest their dreams and build their desired lives.

For network marketers, expressing your true self is a powerful tool for building authentic connections and relationships. You attract like-minded individuals who resonate with your values and beliefs by being genuine and authentic to yourself, leading to more meaningful connections and tremendous success in your business endeavors.

In conclusion, expressing your true self is a journey of self-discovery and self-acceptance. It is about embracing yourself and allowing yourself to shine brightly. So, stop dreaming and start living by expressing your true self in all that you do.

Taking Risks and Embracing Change.

We often choose to play it safe or take a leap of faith. During these moments of decision, we truly discover who we are and what we are capable of. Taking risks and embracing change is terrifying but essential for personal growth and self-awareness.

Taking risks is necessary for those on a journey of self-discovery and seeking truth. It allows us to break free from our comfort zones and challenge ourselves in ways we never thought possible. By embracing change, we open ourselves up to new possibilities and opportunities for growth. We learn more about ourselves and our potential through these challenges and changes.

Dreamers understand the importance of taking risks and embracing change to deepen their practice and connect with their true selves. Dreamers break through barriers and reach new levels of awareness and enlightenment by stepping into the unknown and facing their fears head-on.

Dreamers are often seen as risk-takers, as they pursue their passions and chase their dreams despite the uncertainties that lie ahead. By embracing change and being open to new possibilities, dreamers turn their visions into reality and create the life they desire.

Network marketers also understand the value of taking risks and embracing change to succeed. Network marketers expand their reach and grow their businesses exponentially by stepping outside their comfort zones and trying new strategies.

In the journey to self-awareness, taking risks and embracing change is essential. Through these actions, we discover our true potential and create the life we have always dreamed of. So, don't be afraid to step into the unknown and embrace change – it just leads you to a life beyond your wildest dreams.

# MANIFESTING YOUR DREAMS
# AND CREATING A LIFE YOU LOVE

Visualizing Your Ideal Future.

To indeed start living the life you desire, it is essential to first visualize your ideal future. This process involves tapping into your deepest desires and dreams and creating a clear picture of what you want your life to look like. By visualizing your ideal future, you are setting a powerful intention for the universe to manifest your dreams into reality.

Visualizing your ideal future is a powerful tool for transformation for those on a journey of self-awareness and personal growth. By envisioning the life you want to live, you are aligning your thoughts and emotions with your goals, making it more likely that you will take inspired action toward achieving them.

For dreamers, visualizing your ideal future is a form of meditation. By sitting in stillness and quieting the mind, you more easily connect with your innermost desires and create a clear vision of what you want to manifest in your life.

For network marketers and those searching for truth, visualizing your ideal future helps you stay focused and motivated on your goals. By regularly visualizing the success you want to achieve, you are programming your subconscious mind to work towards making it a reality.

In the realm of self-help and acceptance, visualizing your ideal future is a powerful tool for self-love and acceptance. By imagining the life you want to live, you are affirming your worthiness of experiencing joy, abundance, and fulfillment.

In conclusion, visualizing your ideal future is a critical step in the journey of self-awareness and personal growth. Creating a clear vision of what you want to manifest in your life sets the stage for the universe to bring your dreams into reality. So, stop dreaming and start living by visualizing your desired life.

Taking Inspired Action Toward Your Goals.

Let's delve into the crucial step of turning your dreams into reality. It's one thing to dream and visualize your goals, but it's another to take inspired action towards achieving them. Without action, dreams remain just that - dreams.

For those on the journey to self-awareness, taking inspired action is a powerful way to align your thoughts, beliefs, and actions towards your goals. It is about stepping out of your comfort zone, pushing past your fears and doubts, and working towards making your dreams a reality.

As a dreamer, you already have a strong self-awareness and clarity about your goals. Now is the time to harness that awareness and channel it into tangible actions. Set clear goals, break them down into smaller steps, and take consistent action towards them. Whether meditating on your goals, visualizing success, or actively networking and building connections, every action brings you closer to your dreams.

For network marketers, inspiring action is critical to building a successful business. It's not just about dreaming of success but about actively engaging with your network, promoting your products or services, and continuously learning and growing in your field. By taking inspired action, you move closer to your goals and inspire others to do the same.

In the journey of self-help and self-acceptance, taking inspired action is a way to show yourself love and respect. It is a way to honor your dreams and desires and commit to making them a reality. So stop dreaming and start living by taking inspired action towards your goals today.

Celebrating Your Successes and Practicing Gratitude.

In the journey to self-awareness, celebrating your successes and practicing gratitude is essential. Let's focus on recognizing and appreciating the milestones you have achieved.

For many of us, it is easy to get lost in the hustle and bustle of everyday life, constantly striving for the next goal without acknowledging how far we have come. By celebrating your successes, big or small, you are boosting your confidence and self-esteem and reinforcing positive behaviors that will lead to even more outstanding achievements in the future.

Practicing gratitude is another critical component of self-awareness. By cultivating a mindset of thankfulness, you shift your focus from what you lack to what you have, fostering a sense of abundance and contentment. This simple practice profoundly impacts your overall well-being and outlook on life.

Whether you are a general reader, someone searching for truth, a dreamer, or a network marketer, celebrating your successes and practicing gratitude in your daily routine helps you on your path to self-discovery and personal growth. By reflecting on your achievements and expressing gratitude for the blessings in your life, you are setting yourself up for a more fulfilling and meaningful existence.

So, stop dreaming and start living by embracing and appreciating the present moment. Celebrate how far you have come, practice gratitude for all you have, and watch as your journey to self-awareness unfolds.

# EMBRACING THE SELF-DISCOVERY JOURNEY

Reflecting on Your Personal Growth.

Reflecting on your personal growth is essential in your journey to self-awareness. It allows you to take a moment to pause and look back on how far you have come, the challenges you have overcome, and the lessons you have learned along the way. This process of self-reflection is incredibly empowering. It helps you better understand yourself and your authentic desires.

For many of us, personal growth is complicated and sometimes painful. It requires us to break free from our comfort zone, face our fears, and confront our limitations. However, when we take the time to reflect on our personal growth, we see the positive changes that have occurred within us. We see how we have become more resilient, compassionate, and self-aware.

This subchapter will explore the importance of reflecting on your personal growth and how it positively impacts your life. Whether you are a general reader, someone searching for truth, a dreamer, or a network marketer, this message is universal. Self-reflection is a powerful tool that helps you stop dreaming and start living a more fulfilling and authentic life.

By accepting yourself as you are and embracing your personal growth journey, you cultivate a sense of inner peace and contentment. You learn to let go of self-doubt and fear instead of focusing on your strengths and accomplishments. So take some time to reflect on your personal growth, celebrate your achievements, and continue moving forward on your journey to self-awareness. Remember, the key to fulfilling life lies in embracing who you are and all you have become.

Connecting with Your Inner Wisdom.

Losing touch with our inner wisdom is accessible in our fast-paced and chaotic world. We often get caught up in external distractions and expectations, leaving little or no time for introspection and self-discovery. However, connecting with your inner wisdom is essential for living a fulfilling and authentic life.

Tapping into your inner wisdom provides valuable insights and guidance for those on a journey of self-awareness and personal growth. This inner knowing is like a compass that helps you navigate life's challenges and decisions with clarity and purpose.

Meditation is one of the most effective ways to connect with your inner wisdom. You access deeper awareness, intuition, and peace by quieting your mind, thoughts, and feelings and tuning into your inner silence. Regular meditation helps cultivate inner peace and clarity, making tapping into your inner wisdom easier when faced with difficult decisions or uncertainties.

Dreamers and network marketers benefit greatly from connecting with their inner wisdom. By listening to your inner voice and trusting your instinct, you make more aligned and authentic choices in your personal and professional life. Your inner wisdom helps you uncover your true passions and purpose, guiding you toward a more fulfilling and meaningful path.

For those searching for truth and self-acceptance, connecting with your inner wisdom is a powerful tool for self-discovery and growth. You cultivate a deeper self-awareness and acceptance by embracing your inner knowing and trusting your intuition. Stop dreaming and start living by connecting with your inner wisdom and embracing the truth of who you are.

Embracing the Process of Self-Improvement.

In the quest for self-improvement, embracing the process rather than focusing solely on the end goal is essential. Self-improvement is not a destination but a journey requiring dedication, patience, and a willingness to grow. Let's delve into the importance of accepting oneself as they are while striving to become the best version of themselves.

For those who are dreamers, network marketers, or individuals searching for truth, this subchapter guides understanding the power of self-awareness and personal growth. It emphasizes the need to stop dreaming and start living by taking actionable steps towards self-improvement.

Self-help is not about changing who you are but accepting yourself as you are while acknowledging areas for growth. By embracing the process of self-improvement, individuals cultivate a more profound sense of self-awareness and fulfillment. This journey requires reflection, introspection, and a commitment to personal development.

Whether you are a dreamer with big aspirations, seeking inner peace, or a network marketer looking to enhance your skills, embracing the process of self-improvement is essential for growth and transformation. By recognizing and accepting your strengths and weaknesses, you embark on a journey toward self-discovery and self-empowerment.

Let's remember that self-improvement is a continuous process requiring dedication and perseverance. Embrace the journey, accept yourself as you are, and watch as you evolve into the best version of yourself.

# THE POWER OF NOW AND LIVING IN THE PRESENT MOMENT

Letting Go of Past Regrets and Future Worries.

In our journey towards self-awareness, one of the biggest obstacles we face is letting go of past regrets and future worries. It is human nature to dwell on the mistakes we have made in the past and to constantly worry about what the future holds. However, this constant focus on the past and future prevents us from truly living in the present moment.

To truly embrace self-awareness, we must learn to let go of the things that no longer serve us. This means forgiving ourselves for past mistakes and releasing the burden of carrying around regrets. It also means letting go of the need to constantly worry about what the future holds. By letting go of past regrets and future worries, we free ourselves from the chains that bind us and allow ourselves to fully live in the present moment.

Meditation is one of the most powerful ways to let go of past regrets and future worries. Meditation lets us quiet the mind, let go of negative thoughts, and focus on the present moment. By welcoming meditation into our daily routine, we learn to release the grip of the past and future and fully embrace the present.

As dreamers and network marketers, it is easy to get caught in the hustle and bustle of day-to-day life. However, we find peace and clarity in our lives by learning to let go of past regrets and future worries. By accepting ourselves as we are and embracing the present moment, we stop dreaming and start living to our fullest potential.

Finding Joy and Contentment in the Present Moment.

Finding joy and contentment in the present moment seems daunting in our fast-paced world of distractions and constant demands for attention. However, it is essential for our peace of mind, well-being, and happiness. Let's explore ways to cultivate mindfulness and presence in our daily lives to fully experience the beauty and wonder of each moment.

One of the first steps in finding joy and contentment in the present moment is to let go of the past and future. Many of us spend our days dwelling on past mistakes or worrying about what the future may hold, causing us to miss out on the beauty and opportunities of the present. By practicing mindfulness and focusing on the here and now, we release these burdens and fully immerse ourselves in the present moment.

Meditation is a powerful tool for building presence and awareness. By taking time each day to sit in stillness and quiet the mind, we learn to be fully present in each moment. Through meditation, we develop a deeper connection to ourselves and the world, allowing us to experience joy and contentment in the simplest moments.

For those who struggle with staying present, mindfulness practices such as deep breathing, slow walking, and mindful eating help bring our attention back to the present moment.

By engaging fully with our senses and physical sensations, we anchor ourselves in the here and now, allowing us to experience joy and contentment in the present moment.

Ultimately, finding joy and contentment in the present moment is a practice that requires patience, self-compassion, and dedication. By cultivating mindfulness and presence in our daily lives, we learn to appreciate the beauty and richness of each moment, leading to a more fulfilling and meaningful life.

Practicing Mindfulness in Everyday Life.

Practicing mindfulness is a powerful tool that helps you achieve self-awareness and live a more fulfilling life. Mindfulness means being fully present and engaged in the moment without judgment or distraction. It allows you to nourish a deeper connection with yourself and the world, leading to greater clarity, peace, and contentment.

Mindfulness is a transformative practice for those constantly dreaming and seeking truth. By bringing your attention to the present moment, you let go of worries about the future and regrets from the past. This allows you to fully experience and appreciate the beauty and opportunities here and now.

Dreamers benefit from incorporating mindfulness into their daily routines. Whether sitting in meditation or doing your daily tasks, being mindful helps you stay centered and focused. It also enables you to become more attuned to your thoughts, emotions, and behaviors, allowing you to make conscious choices that align with your true desires and values.

For network marketers, practicing mindfulness is especially valuable. By cultivating present-moment awareness, you better connect with others, build authentic relationships, and make more informed decisions. Mindfulness also helps you stay grounded in the face of challenges and setbacks, allowing you to navigate the ups and downs of the business world with grace and resilience.

Practicing mindfulness in everyday life is a critical step in self-awareness. By incorporating it into your daily routine, you stop dreaming and live a more authentic, fulfilling life. Accept yourself as you are, embrace the present moment, and watch as your true potential unfolds.

# CONCLUSIONS

We are already okay as we are; all more we get and become is simply an acknowledgment bonus from life.

We spend so much time dreaming about what we want to be, what we want to have, and what we want to do. We dream about the perfect job, the perfect partner, the perfect house, and the perfect life. But what if we stopped dreaming and just accepted ourselves as we are?

What if we stopped trying to be someone we're not and just embraced who we are? What if we stopped trying to change our bodies and just loved them the way they were? What if we stopped trying to be perfect and just accepted our flaws?

If we stopped dreaming and accepted ourselves as we were, we would be much happier. We would be free from the pressure to be someone we're not. We would be free from the need to constantly compare ourselves to others. We would be free to just be ourselves.

Of course, it's not always easy to accept ourselves as we are. We all have flaws and insecurities. But if we focus on our strengths and what makes us unique, we can learn to love ourselves for who we are.

So, if you're feeling down, I encourage you to stop dreaming and accept yourself. You are already okay as you are; all more you get and become is simply an acknowledgment bonus from life.

Here are some tips on how to accept yourself as you are:

1. Focus on your strengths. Everyone has strengths and weaknesses. Please make a list of your strengths and focus on them. This will help you to see the good in yourself.

2. Be kind to yourself. We are all our own worst critics. We need to be kind to ourselves and forgive ourselves for our mistakes.

3. Love yourself unconditionally. We must love ourselves for who we are, our flaws, and all. We must accept ourselves for who we are, not who we think we should be.

4. Surround yourself with positive people. The people we surround ourselves with have a significant impact on our self-esteem. Make sure to surround yourself with positive people who love and support you.

5. Practice self-care. Self-care is critical for our physical and mental health. Take care of yourself by eating healthy, talking positively, exercising, watching positive TV programs, and getting enough sleep.

Accepting yourself as you are is a journey, not a destination. It takes time and effort. But it is worth it. Accept yourself as you are, and you will be free to live your life to the fullest.

With all my love and support, Andrea.

# BIBLIOGRAPHY

Scarsi, Andrea: Happy To Be Happy
Scarsi, Andrea: The Secret Of Meditation
Scarsi, Andrea: The Art of Worrying
Scarsi, Andrea: Romance Ain't Love Pollution

# ABOUT THE AUTHOR

Dr. Andrea Scarsi, also known as Swami Prem Sandesh, is a master of meditation who defines himself as a mystic, metaphysician, author, musician, and wellness coach when he uses his works to share a dimension of being, lifestyle, and knowledge, founded on the communion with the absolute.

Born in Venice, Italy, in 1955, he began practicing yoga and spiritism and experimenting with telepathy at fifteen. He contacts alien and transdimensional entities at eighteen, following a near-death experience. At twenty-four, on his first trip to India, he finds himself a vegetarian and in the world of meditation led by India and the Spiritual Master Osho, receiving Sandesh as a new name, which he wears in specific environments.

He has often traveled, especially to India, residing for long periods also in Nepal, the Philippines, Brazil, and Buddhist Southeast Asia: Japan, Thailand, Sri Lanka, Hong Kong, Laos, China, and Tibet, exploring local places and cultures, meeting people and participating in ritual and religious practices.

Over time, he delved into various meditative techniques for awakening consciousness, energy rebalancing, and personal evolution, which he practices and teaches. He studied philosophy, earned a doctorate in metaphysical science, and various diplomas such as Holistic Life Coach, Reiki Grand Master, Master of Crystals, Shamanism, Meditation and Massage and Wellness Coach.

He's into cellular nutrition, holistic wellness, and Network Marketing. In 1991, he married Krisana, and they now live in Venice, Italy. Reach him at andrea.scarsi@yahoo.com.

# BOOKS BY ANDREA SCARSI

Answers For The Soul: Fragments of Eternal Wisdom
Blessings! Dedicated to Osho
Extraterrestrial Channeling: Alien Abduction Syndrome
Happy To Be Happy: The Grand Manual Of Happiness
Home Sweet Home Staging: Easy Is Right
How To Ask A Woman Out: Gentlemen Only
Indigo Crystal Rainbow and Diamond: Tell Themselves
Journey To The Underworld: First Level Shamanic Procedures Manual
Make Your Own Vineyard: Ex Vite Vita
O Iguana! My Iguana! Herbivore is Beautiful
Pearls of Wisdom: Tales of Ordinary Metaphysics
Reiki First Degree Manual
Reiki Second Degree Manual
Reiki Third Degree Manual
Romance Ain't Love Pollution: Romance Will Never Die
Seeds Of Enlightenment: The Buddha Within
Tarot Reading Essentials: The New Basic Meaning Manual
The Art of Persuasion: Achieve Your Goals Ethically
The Art of Worrying: How to Enter and Exit it at Will
The Master And The Assassin: An Ordinary Zen Story
The Secret Of Meditation: The Inner Dimension
The Secret Of Metaphysical Science: Our Eternal Journey Through Infinite
The Silence of The Absolute: Satsang with Sandesh
Vegetarian Cuisine: Reasons Objections Recipes
Walking The Dogs: A Dialogue A Manual
Zen The Sense Of Nonsense: Anecdotes For Synaptic Deprogramming

# MANTRAS BY ANDREA SCARSI (SANDESH)

Mantras Mahamantras
The Mantra Experiment
The Mantra Way
Om Namo Supernova
Amāvasya
Lingamananda

A mantra is a verbal being that acts as a bridge between the human and the divine. It carries our prayer, thankfulness, and gratitude. It is an entity in its own right. When we recite or sing it to communicate with the superior dimension, in addition to words and sound, we also employ intention, energy, devotion, and focus. All this raises us immediately. It increases our emotional state and makes us touch God. A mantra is an introspective event turning to the multiple aspects of the One by evoking its symbolic names: Shiva, Brahma, Vishnu, Ganesha, Laxmi, Saraswati, Gurudev, and Shanti, names representing the infinite manifestation of the cosmic cycle.

They are magic formulas for amending the universal present, resolving the apparent fragmentation, and recreating the union of consciousness with what is. A mantra is to be recited and sung without interruption to convey the intact message, and breathing comes between recitations. Let's get lost in the mantra and let the vehicle, the human, and the divine become one. That's the power of the mantra. We recite it and go deeper until melting what we were before, our intention, recitation, sound, and collective energy, and manifesting unity once again, the yoga of consciousness, the absolute presence, whose supreme name is Om.

50

You've reached the end of
*Stop Dreaming: Accept Yourself As You Are.*
Thank You for reading.
Andrea Scarsi